THE POWER OF REGULAR EXERCISE

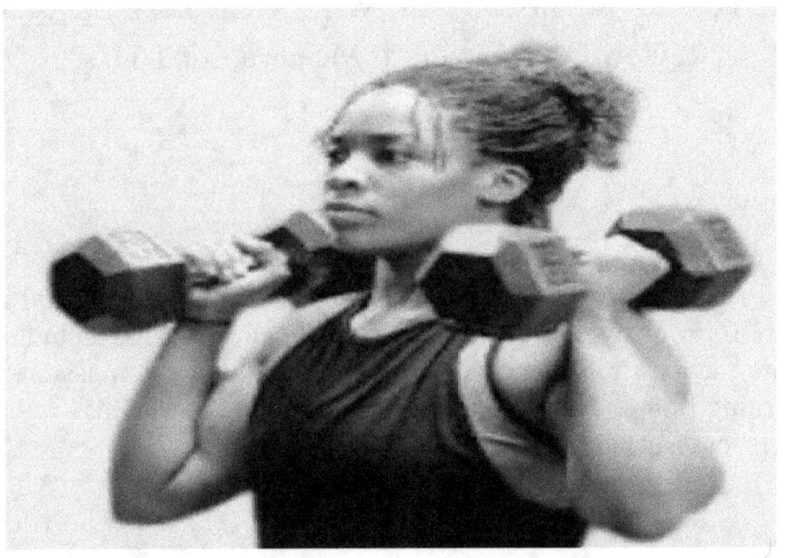

How Physical Activity Boosts Your Overall Health

Dr. Sophia Wellness

THANK YOU FOR CHOOSING US.

We Appreciate Your Kind Support And We Hope You Got Something Out Of It.

If You Enjoy This Book, It Will Be Great To <u>Leave a Review On Amazon</u>. It Means a Lot To Us.

ENJOY OUR SERVICES.

Published by Harmony House Publishers

Table of Contents

INTRODUCTION

Unleashing the Potential of Exercise

Have you ever been astounded by the remarkable changes that people experience when they start a regular workout regimen? Maybe you've seen someone lose weight, get stronger, or exude contagious energy that seemed to come from deep inside. Exercise can transform not only our bodies but also our overall well-being, it's almost miraculous.

Imagine a scenario in which you could access this revolutionary force. Imagine a world where engaging in regular physical activity may provide you with more energy, stronger muscles, better cardiovascular health, and improved mental wellness. You can access this planet.

Let me tell you a story to set the scene for our adventure together. Meet Sarah, a cheerful woman who battled low energy, erratic moods, and a general sense of unhappiness in her life. She discovered that she had fallen into the trap of a sedentary lifestyle and spent the entire day hardly getting out of her computer chair.

Sarah decided to take charge of her health and well-being one day. She began to include frequent exercise in her schedule, starting with simple actions like going to a nearby yoga class and taking brisk walks during her lunch break. Over time, a remarkable event transpired. A newfound sense of vigor started to flow through Sarah's veins. Her energy levels increased dramatically, her mood improved, and she gained fresh mental and physical fortitude.

There are innumerable examples of how exercise can change lives, and Sarah's tale is just one of them. It affects every part of who we are and affects changes that are not just physical. Our cardiovascular health, the way our muscles look, our flexibility and balance, and even our cognitive function can all be dramatically improved by exercise. The advantages are simply amazing.

Let's study the science of exercise and all the different ways it might improve your health. We will learn the techniques for maximizing the potential of your body, from cardiovascular fitness to developing strength, flexibility, and balance. But it goes further than that. We'll also shed some light on how important exercise is for managing stress, improving mood, and maintaining mental health.

You will discover how to personalize your workout regimen, get over difficulties, and keep consistency with useful guidance, expert insights, and doable techniques. We'll talk about typical problems and provide pointers for getting help and taking responsibility. Together, we'll discover exercise's transformational potential and give you the tools you need to live a healthier, happier, and more fulfilling life.

Are you prepared to start this voyage, then? Let's maximize exercise's potential and open up a world of opportunities for your physical and emotional well-being. Prepare to be amazed as you learn about "The Power of Regular Exercise: How Physical Activity Boosts Your Overall Health."

The transformative impact of exercise on our bodies and minds

Regular exercise transforms our bodies and minds, opening up a world of advantages that go far beyond physical health. Our bodies react to physical activity in amazing ways, undergoing beneficial changes that improve our general well-being.

Physically, exercise builds muscle, strengthens the heart, and increases endurance. Our capacity to handle daily chores with ease and energy increases as we become more resilient. Our bodies get stronger, more energized, and more capable of handling the stresses of daily life.

But exercise has benefits that go beyond the physical. Our brains release endorphins during physical exertion, also known as the "feel-good" hormones. Our mood is improved by these endorphins, which also lessen tension and increase feelings of well-being and happiness. Exercise turns into a potent instrument for fighting depression and anxiety, providing a simple and effective technique to enhance our mental health.

Additionally, exercise improves cognitive function by helping us focus better, remember things better, and be more creative. It enhances neural connections and encourages the development of new neurons, which improves our capacity for thought, learning, and problem-solving. Regular exercise has been associated with increased mental clarity, increased productivity, and a higher level of mental alertness.

Exercise has a profoundly transforming effect on our life that goes beyond the physical and mental spheres. Our confidence increases as we see how much stronger our bodies are becoming. We gain a more favorable perception of ourselves and a renewed sense of self-confidence. As a result, we develop greater resiliency and are better able to meet challenges and get through roadblocks.

Additionally, exercise fosters community and social interaction. We can meet people who share our passion for health and wellness by taking part in team sports, participating in group activities, or signing up for fitness programs. These social ties provide assistance, inspiration, and a sense of community, developing a deeper sense of satisfaction and meaning.

In essence, physical activity can improve our physical and mental health as well as our general quality of life. It opens the door to a life that is more energetic, empowered, and content. By accepting exercise's transforming effects, we open up a world of opportunities and put ourselves on a path to long-term health, happiness, and self-discovery.

A personal story:

Overcoming obstacles through the power of regular exercise

Let me share with you a personal experience that exemplifies the positive effects of consistent exercise. Meet Mark, a middle-aged man who had been experiencing feelings of lack of energy, self-doubt, and unhappiness in his life. He sensed himself caught in a downward spiral and realized something had to happen.

Mark decided to include regular exercise in his daily regimen with a glimmer of hope. It was tough at first. He ran across physical obstacles and questioned his ability to persevere. Mark persisted nonetheless, driven by a desire for a better life.

Something amazing happened as soon as he started moving about. Mark started to feel stronger and more alive than before. He could feel his body getting stronger and his energy levels rising with each session. But more than the physical changes, he was astounded by the improvement in his mental and emotional health.

Mark found that going to the gym regularly allowed him to escape the stress and pressures of daily life. His spirit was lifted, his mind was clear, and he felt better as he exercised. Exercise evolved into his form of therapy, allowing him to let go of repressed feelings, lessen anxiety, and find comfort in the rhythm of movement.

Mark also experienced a renewed sense of self-belief thanks to the effectiveness of regular exercise. His confidence grew as he cleared obstacles and hit little milestones. He started to think of himself as strong and capable, not limited by his past setbacks.

Beyond Mark's personal life, exercise had a transforming impact. His renewed energy and optimistic outlook started to spread to other aspects of his life. He improved his work output, relationship commitment, and openness to new options. The once insurmountable challenges now proved to be stepping stones for growth and personal development.

Mark's experience serves as a potent reminder that regular exercise is about more than just maintaining physical health; it is also a means of fostering self-awareness, resiliency, and transformation. We may overcome challenges, overcome constraints, and realize our full potential by embracing the power of regular exercise.

So keep in mind Mark's motivational narrative when you're struggling with bodily issues, looking for mental stability, or desiring a feeling of purpose that has been reignited. Utilize the power of consistent exercise and watch as it catalyzes empowerment, personal growth, and living a life beyond your wildest expectations.

CHAPTER 1

THE SCIENCE BEHIND EXERCISE: HOW IT ENHANCES YOUR WELL-BEING

Exercise improves your general well-being through a surprising variety of processes, according to scientists. Beyond the obvious physical changes, exercise sets off a chain of beneficial physiological reactions in your body and mind.

Your heart pumps more oxygen-rich blood to your muscles while you exercise because your heart rate quickens. Your cardiovascular fitness increases thanks to this procedure, which also strengthens and increases the effectiveness of your heart muscle. Regular exercise over time can lower blood pressure, lower your resting heart rate, and minimize your chance of developing cardiovascular problems.

Exercise is essential for controlling your metabolism and body weight. Calorie burning is a key factor in weight management and preventing excess weight gain. Your metabolism is boosted, which results in more effective energy use and could support weight loss attempts. Additionally, exercise promotes the preservation of lean muscle mass, which is essential for preserving a healthy body composition.

Exercise has a significant impact on your mental and emotional health in addition to its physical advantages. Endorphins, brain neurotransmitters known as "feel-good" hormones, are stimulated to be released. These endorphins induce emotions of joy, lessen stress, and lessen anxiety and depressive symptoms. Regular exercise can have a positive impact on your mood, self-esteem, and mental clarity, acting as a natural antidepressant.

Exercise is linked to better brain health and cognitive performance. Increased blood flow to the brain, which brings oxygen and nutrients that support neuronal growth and improve cognitive function, is the result of physical activity. Studies have demonstrated that regular exercise can improve cognitive function in general, including memory and attention span. Even the risk of neurodegenerative illnesses like Alzheimer's and dementia might be lowered as a result.

Additionally, physical activity encourages the release of several neurotransmitters and growth factors in the brain, including brain-derived neurotrophic factor (BDNF). These compounds encourage the growth of new neurons and fortify brain connections, which promote learning, problem-solving abilities, and mental toughness.

Exercise has advantages that go beyond its immediate physiological impact. Regular physical activity can improve the quality of your sleep, strengthen your immune system, and increase your overall vigor and productivity. In addition, it can provide you with a sense of achievement, discipline, and personal pleasure, all of which help you think positively and feel better overall.

We are better able to incorporate physical activity into our lives by making educated decisions when we understand the science behind exercise. We may maximize our well-being, live healthier lives, and reach the full potential of our physical and mental capabilities by taking advantage of the tremendous impacts that exercise has on our bodies and brains. So let's embrace the benefits of exercise that science has proven and start along the path to a healthier, happier, and more contented life.

Understanding the physiological changes that occur during exercise

Your body experiences several amazing physiological changes while you work out. These adjustments are essential for raising general health, increasing fitness, and maximizing performance. Let's examine the main physiological changes brought on by exercise:

Your heart rate increases as you begin exercising to keep up with the increased demand for oxygen and nutrients to be delivered to your working muscles. This faster heartbeat makes it easier to deliver oxygenated blood and effectively remove waste.

- **Improved Cardiorespiratory System:** Regular exercise makes your cardiovascular and respiratory systems more effective. Your heart muscle gets stronger, increasing the amount of blood it can pump with each beat. As a result, the stroke volume increases, allowing your heart to pump more oxygen-rich blood to your muscles with each contraction. Exercise also helps to build up the breathing muscles, which enhances lung capacity and oxygen absorption.

- **Better Blood Circulation:** Exercise encourages angiogenesis, the process of creating new blood vessels. This wider network of blood vessels improves blood flow to your muscles, organs, and tissues, facilitating the supply of nutrients and the elimination of waste. Enhanced circulation also aids in controlling body temperature when exercising.

- **Muscle adaptations:** Your muscles undergo several adaptations as a result of regular exercise. As your muscles adapt to the increasing strain during resistance training, they get stronger and more toned. Your muscles can utilize oxygen more effectively and maintain sustained activity thanks to endurance activities that increase their oxidative capacity. Strength, stamina, and general muscle performance are all enhanced as a result of these adaptations.

- **Increased Oxygen Consumption:** As you work out, your body uses more oxygen to produce the necessary amount of energy. Your breathing speed and depth increase in response, enabling you to inhale more oxygen and exhale more carbon dioxide. Your muscles are fed by this increased oxygen demand, which also increases energy production.

- **Elevated Metabolism:** Exercise speeds up your metabolism, which raises your energy consumption. During exercise and at rest, your body gets more effective at burning calories. Maintaining a healthy body weight and assisting with weight loss are both possible with regular exercise.

- Endorphins, which are responsible for the "feel-good" sensation and pain relief, are released as a result of exercise, among other hormones. Growth hormone, which aids in muscle growth and repair, is also stimulated during exercise. Exercise can also aid in regulating the hormones that affect metabolism, hunger, and stress response.

Understanding these physiological alterations that occur during exercise enables you to grasp the profound effects that exercise has on your body. By exercising regularly, you can improve your cardiovascular health, muscle strength and endurance, oxygen use, and metabolism in general. These adjustments help to boost energy levels, fitness, and overall wellness of the body and mind. So put on your shoes, get moving, and unleash the incredible physiological benefits of exercise in your body.

Unveiling the benefits of exercise for physical and mental health

Exercise regularly is a potent instrument that has a wealth of advantages for your physical and emotional well-being. Exercise has a profoundly favorable impact on your health, whether you choose to do it vigorously (like running or weightlifting) or moderately (like brisk walking). Let's examine the impressive advantages of exercise:

Physical Fitness:

- **Increased Cardiovascular Fitness:** Exercise makes your heart stronger, increasing its effectiveness and lowering your risk of heart disease. It promotes a healthier cardiovascular system by enhancing blood circulation and lowering blood pressure.

- **Weight management:** By burning calories and gaining lean muscle mass, regular exercise helps maintain healthy body weight. Both weight gain and fat loss are prevented by it.
- Strength and endurance in the muscles are increased through exercise, which also tones the muscles. Injury prevention and joint health are supported by strong muscles.
- **Bone Density Increased:** Weight-bearing activities like walking and weightlifting encourage bone growth and increase bone density, which lowers the risk of osteoporosis.
- Exercise improves flexibility, balance, and coordination, which promotes greater physical function overall and lowers the chance of accidents and injuries.

Mental Wellness:

- **Enhancement of Mood:** Endorphins, the brain's natural "feel-good" chemicals, are released during exercise and help to improve mood, lower stress levels, and lessen the symptoms of anxiety and melancholy.
- **Increased Energy and Vitality:** Regular physical exercise enhances your general vitality, combats fatigue, and increases your energy levels, making you feel more energized and alert.

- **Enhanced Cognitive Function:** Exercise improves cognitive function, such as memory, attention, and problem-solving skills, by boosting neuroplasticity, increasing blood flow to the brain, and supporting brain health.
- **Stress Reduction:** Engaging in physical activity will help you release tension and enhance your capacity to handle obstacles in daily life.
- **Enhanced Self-Esteem and Body Image:** Regular exercise can develop a good self-perception by enhancing self-esteem, body image, and self-confidence.

Generally Speaking:

- **higher Sleep:** Exercise encourages higher sleep quality, making it easier to get to sleep and stay asleep for longer periods.
- Living an active lifestyle is linked to a longer lifespan and a lower risk of developing chronic diseases.
- **Improved Immune Function:** Regular exercise helps to build immune function, which lowers the chance of contracting common illnesses and improves general health.

You can reap a plethora of advantages for your physical and mental health by including exercise in your regimen. It catalyzes good transformation, supporting overall wellness and making life happier and healthier. So put on your running shoes, look for things you like to do, and embrace the amazing things exercise can do for your mind, body, and general quality of life.

CHAPTER 2

CARDIOVASCULAR FITNESS: STRENGTHENING YOUR HEART AND CIRCULATORY SYSTEM

Cardiovascular fitness, sometimes referred to as aerobic fitness or cardiovascular endurance, is the capacity of your heart, lungs, and circulatory system to effectively supply oxygen-rich blood to your muscles when you are physically active. It is an essential part of general fitness and helps to keep the cardiovascular system in good shape. The value of cardiovascular fitness and how it supports your heart and circulatory system will be discussed.

- **Heart Strength:** Cardiovascular exercise regularly strengthens your heart muscle, improving blood pumping efficiency. Running, cycling, and swimming are examples of activities that raise your heart rate. As you practice these sports, your heart responds by getting more powerful. With more power, it may pump more blood with each beat, lowering the resting heart rate and improving circulation both at rest and during physical activity.

- **Improved Blood Flow:** Cardiovascular exercise improves your body's blood flow. It causes blood vessels to swell, making it possible for your working muscles to receive oxygen and nutrients more effectively. The improved muscle performance and decreased risk of weariness are both a result of the increased blood flow, which also improves the clearance of waste products from your muscles, such as carbon dioxide.

- **Blood Pressure:** Cardiovascular exercise regularly can help reduce blood pressure levels. Blood flow resistance is decreased by physical activity because it causes blood vessels to expand and become more flexible. As a result, less pressure is placed on the arterial walls, which lowers both systolic (the top number) and diastolic blood pressure. The stress on the heart is lessened by decreased blood pressure, which also lowers the risk of cardiovascular disease.

- **Enhanced Endurance:** By increasing your cardiovascular fitness, you can maintain physical activity for longer periods without getting tired. Regular aerobic exercise improves the effectiveness of your respiratory system, your blood's ability to deliver oxygen, and your body's ability to use oxygen. You may carry out daily work and take on more strenuous physical activities with increased ease and endurance thanks to these adaptations.

- **Reduced chance of Cardiovascular disorders:** Cardiovascular disorders like coronary artery disease, heart attacks, and strokes are linked to a lower chance of development when regular exercise is done. It encourages ideal blood lipid profiles, lowers the accumulation of arterial plaque, and aids in maintaining healthy cholesterol levels. Regular physical activity can also reduce the risk of type 2 diabetes, a key risk factor for heart disease, by regulating blood sugar levels and enhancing insulin sensitivity.

Exercises that improve your heart and circulation system should include aerobics. Aim for 75 minutes of strong aerobic exercise, 150 minutes of moderate aerobic exercise, or a combination of the two every week. To make your cardiovascular workouts more pleasurable and sustainable, choose activities you will enjoy. You can maintain a healthier heart, improve circulation, and enjoy a host of advantages associated with a robust and effective cardiovascular system by increasing your cardiovascular fitness.

Exploring the Role of aerobic exercises in improving cardiovascular health

By supporting effective oxygen distribution throughout the body, strengthening the heart and lungs, and engaging in aerobic activity, cardiovascular health can be significantly improved. These activities, also called cardio or cardiovascular ones, raise your heart rate and speed up your breathing, which has several positive effects on your cardiovascular system. Let's examine how aerobic exercise specifically enhances cardiovascular health:

Exercises that challenge and build the heart's muscles are known as aerobics. Your heart has to work harder to pump oxygenated blood to your working muscles as you perform activities like brisk walking, jogging, cycling, or dancing. Regular cardiovascular exercise allows the heart muscle to adapt and strengthen over time. Lower resting heart rates and improved cardiac function are both effects of a stronger heart's ability to pump blood more effectively.

1. **Enhancing Lung Function:** By expanding the capacity of your lungs, aerobic exercises also enhance lung function. When you engage in aerobic exercise, your breathing becomes deeper and faster, which develops

and increases the efficiency of your respiratory muscles. Better oxygen absorption and carbon dioxide expulsion are made possible by these improved lung functions, which optimize the oxygenation of your muscles and organs.

2. **Improved Circulation of Blood:** Regular aerobic exercise increases blood flow throughout the body. Cardio exercises cause the blood vessels to enlarge, which increases the blood flow to the muscles and organs. The tissues receive oxygen and nutrients more quickly because of the increased circulation, which also more efficiently removes waste materials like carbon dioxide. Improved blood circulation also lowers the chance of developing cardiovascular diseases and supports appropriate blood pressure levels.

3. **Lowering Cholesterol Levels:** It has been demonstrated that aerobic exercise raises levels of high-density lipoprotein (HDL), or "good" cholesterol. Low-density lipoprotein (LDL), or "bad" cholesterol, is removed from the bloodstream with the aid of HDL cholesterol. Aerobic exercise helps to improve HDL cholesterol and lower LDL cholesterol, which results in a healthier lipid profile and a lower risk of heart disease.

4. Weight management and body composition control can be achieved with regular aerobic exercise. By burning calories, these activities can aid in weight loss and weight maintenance. As excess weight puts an additional

burden on the heart and raises the risk of developing heart disease and other disorders, maintaining healthy body weight is crucial for cardiovascular health.

5. **Risk Reduction for Chronic Diseases:** Aerobic exercise has been linked to a reduced risk of several chronic diseases. Cardiovascular exercise regularly helps lower the risk of diseases like coronary artery disease, stroke, type 2 diabetes, and several cancers. Exercises that improve cardiovascular health also enhance insulin sensitivity, blood sugar regulation, and metabolic health in general.

Aim for at least 150 minutes of moderate-intensity aerobic activity or 75 minutes of vigorous-intensity aerobic activity each week to reap the benefits of aerobic exercises for cardiovascular health. To keep a routine interesting and enduring, pick activities you enjoy doing.

Effective strategies for boosting endurance and enhancing heart function

Key objectives for those wishing to increase their cardiovascular fitness include increasing endurance and improving heart health. You may improve your levels of endurance and encourage a healthy heart by putting into practice effective tactics. Here are some tactics to take into account:

1. **Gradual Progression:** Begin by progressively lengthening and intensifying your exercises. This enables your body to adapt and gradually increase its endurance. As your fitness improves, start with shorter exercises at a comfortable level and gradually increase the time or intensity.

2. Exercises that test your circulatory system and raise your heart rate are referred to as cardiovascular exercises. Running, cycling, swimming, or utilizing cardio devices like the elliptical or rowing machine are some examples of these workouts. Set a weekly goal of 75 minutes of intense aerobic activity or 150 minutes of moderate aerobic exercise.

3. Consider using interval training in your routines. This entails switching back and forth between intense workouts and active recuperation. For instance, you may sprint for 30 seconds, followed by a minute of walking or jogging, and then repeat the process. By enhancing both aerobic and anaerobic endurance via interval training, you may push yourself to the limit and raise your cardiovascular fitness.

4. By engaging in a range of cardiovascular exercises, you may engage various muscle groups and put your body through several challenges. In addition to preventing

boredom, cross-training increases overall endurance and lowers the chance of overuse injuries. To add variety to your routines, including activities like swimming, cycling, dancing, or group fitness programs.

5. Exercises for strength training should be included in your regimen regularly. You can retain appropriate form and endurance during cardiovascular exercises by strengthening your muscles, which support and shield your joints. Aim for two to three sessions of strength training each week, with an emphasis on the main muscle groups.

6. **Frequency and Consistency:** Frequency is important for increasing endurance. Aim to do cardiovascular activities three to five times a week, minimum. Regularity enables your body to adapt and develop over time while laying a solid aerobic foundation.

7. Maintain a well-balanced diet that gives you the energy and nutrition you need for your exercises. Drink enough water. A healthy diet helps with endurance and overall performance. Additionally, drink plenty of water before, during, and after exercise to improve heart health and avoid dehydration, which may reduce endurance.

8. **Rest and recovery:** Give your body enough time between exercises to heal. Days of rest are essential for both general and muscular regeneration. To avoid overtraining and burnout, pay attention to your body and change the amount of time or intensity you spend exercising as necessary.

CHAPTER 3

BUILDING STRENGTH: SCULPTING MUSCLES AND ENHANCING PERFORMANCE

1. Strength training is a crucial part of staying physically fit overall and can have a big impact on how well your muscles grow and perform. There are efficient methods to help you sculpt muscles and improve performance, whether your goal is to raise your strength for sports endeavors or simply to improve your physique. Let's examine some essential methods for enhancing your strength:

2. **Resistance Training:** Add resistance training to your daily exercise regimen. You might do this by applying resistance via free weights, exercise machines, resistance bands, or even your body weight. Concentrate on compound movements like squats, deadlifts, bench presses, and pull-ups that concurrently work for many muscular groups. Lifting weights or resistance should be gradually increased to keep your muscles guessing and encourage strength increases.

3. Put the idea of gradual overload into practice during your workouts. The demands placed on your muscles

will gradually increase as a result. By raising the weight, repetitions, sets, or intensity of your exercises, you can attain it. Your muscles adapt and become stronger to handle the greater demands when you challenge them regularly.

4. Pay attention to good form and technique when performing strength training activities. By doing this, you may be confident that you're efficiently targeting the desired muscle groups while lowering your chance of damage. Consider working with a professional personal trainer who can mentor you and offer criticism if you're unsure of the proper form.

5. **Exercise Variety:** Include a range of exercises to work on various muscle groups and prevent plateauing. By constantly switching up your workouts, you test your muscles in new ways and encourage additional muscle growth. Consider including exercises for the legs, chest, back, shoulders, arms, and core, as well as for all the major muscle groups.

6. **Adequate Rest and Recovery:** Give your muscles enough time between sessions to heal. Muscle fibers are damaged during strength training, and they are repaired and made stronger during recovery. Aim for a minimum of 48 hours between workouts that target the same muscle group. Prioritize getting enough sleep, eating well, and staying hydrated on rest days to aid in muscle growth and recovery.

7. Maintain a balanced diet that contains the nutrients required for muscle growth and repair. Consume enough protein to assist the production of new muscle tissue. Your meals should contain a variety of fruits, vegetables, nutritious grains, and lean protein sources. To maximize your performance overall and muscle function, stay hydrated.

8. **Consistency and Persistence:** It takes time and consistency to develop strength. Aim for two to three workouts each week and incorporate strength training into your normal exercise program. Maintain your commitment to your workouts and accept the idea of making slow, steady development. Gaining strength requires perseverance and consistent effort.

9. **Track Your Progress:** Keep tabs on your progress during strength training to keep track of your advancements and maintain motivation. Keep a journal of your workouts, including the weights and reps, and occasionally evaluate your strength by measuring your one-rep maximum or using other techniques.

Discovering the importance of strength training for overall fitness

A crucial part of total fitness is strength training, which frequently complements cardiovascular exercise. While cardio exercises have several advantages for cardiovascular health, strength training has particular advantages that make it a valuable component of a well-rounded fitness regimen. You can gain a variety of advantages from strength training that goes beyond simply adding muscle to your body. Let's examine why strength training is crucial for general fitness:

1. Strength training involves resistance exercises that target particular muscle parts, pushing them to grow stronger. This results in an increase in muscle strength and endurance. Exercises that gradually increase resistance or weight enhance the growth and adaptation of muscle fibers. This increases muscle strength and endurance, making it easier for you to carry out daily chores and lowering your chance of developing muscular imbalances or weakness.

2. Strength exercise has a favorable effect on your metabolism, increasing it. Strength training improves lean muscle mass, which causes you to burn more calories even while you're at rest. Having a greater

metabolic rate can help you maintain a healthy weight and encourage fat loss, which can be advantageous for your weight management and body composition goals.

3. Strength training is essential for maintaining and enhancing bone density. It also helps prevent injuries. Your bones experience stress through weight-bearing exercises like lifting weights or using resistance machines, which encourages them to grow stronger and denser. For those who are susceptible to osteoporosis or age-related bone loss, this is especially crucial. Stronger bones promote overall bone health and lower the incidence of fractures.

4. Strengthening the muscles around your joints helps to increase joint stability and lowers the chance of injuries, which improves joint function. Strength training activities encourage the growth of connective tissues that support your joints during movement, such as tendons and ligaments. This is especially advantageous for people who have joint issues or are healing from accidents.

5. **Daily Activities and Functional Fitness:** Strength training improves functional fitness, which is the capacity to carry out tasks of daily living with comfort and effectiveness. You'll find it simpler to lift and carry goods, climb stairs, complete household tasks, and partake in leisure activities as your general muscle

strength increases. This results in an improved quality of life and more independence with daily activities.

6. Strength training is a crucial part of improving athletic performance, regardless of the sport or activity you engage in. Power, speed, agility, and general physical performance are all improved. You can improve your performance in sports, leisure activities, and even in reaching your fitness objectives, like running faster or jumping higher, by gaining strength.

7. Strength training activities target certain muscles that are important for maintaining good posture and correct body alignment. This improves body mechanics and posture. Your posture will improve, lowering your risk of back pain and improving your general body mechanics. This is made possible by strengthening the muscles in your core, back, and hips. Better stability and balance are further benefits.

8. **Mental and Emotional Well-Being:** Strength exercising regularly can improve your mental and emotional health. Endorphins, which are natural mood boosters, are released during exercise, especially strength training. It can lessen the signs of anxiety, despair, and stress, encouraging a happier perspective and greater mental wellness.

Strength training doesn't have to result in bulking up or turning into a bodybuilder for you to incorporate into your fitness regimen. It aims to enhance your general health, functionality, and fitness.

Effective techniques and exercises for building and toning muscles

Resistance training exercises and efficient methods that target particular muscle groups are combined to build and tone muscles. You may increase muscle growth and get a better-contoured physique by combining these methods into your training regimen. These efficient methods and exercises for developing and toning muscles are listed below:

1. Exercises with several joints that simultaneously work various muscle groups are known as compound exercises. These workouts are very helpful in increasing muscle mass and general strength. Squats, deadlifts, bench presses, overhead presses, and pull-ups are a few examples. Compound exercises allow you to work for numerous muscular groups in a single action, which promotes effective muscle growth.

2. **Progressive Overload:** A key component of the muscular building is progressive overload. It entails progressively putting more stress on your muscles over time. By increasing the weight, repetitions, sets, or intensity of your exercises, you can create a progressive

overload. Your muscles adapt and become stronger when you constantly put them through hardship.

3. **Exercises in Isolation:** Isolation exercises target particular muscle groups, allowing you to concentrate on building and toning those parts of your body. Bicep curls, tricep extensions, lateral raises, and calf raises are a few examples. Utilizing isolation exercises in your regimen can help you define and shape the right muscles, giving you a toned and balanced appearance.

4. **High-Intensity Interval Training (HIIT)** is a type of exercise that alternates quick bursts of vigorous activity with rest intervals. This kind of exercise promotes fat loss and muscle endurance gains. Bodyweight movements like burpees, squat leaps, and mountain climbers are frequently used in HIIT workouts. You can increase your metabolism, burn calories, and tone your muscles by including HIIT in your program.

5. **Circuit Training:** In circuit training, several exercises are performed one after the other with little rest in between. It works a variety of muscle groups while maintaining a high heart rate, which has both cardiovascular and strength advantages. By choosing a selection of resistance workouts and adding aerobic exercises like jumping jacks or skipping rope, you may design your circuit.

6. **Dropsets and supersets:** In a superset, two exercises for various muscle groups are done back-to-back without a

break. Adding a back row exercise to a chest press, for instance. By increasing the tension and stress on your muscles, this approach encourages muscle development and toning. Dropsets entail working through an exercise set until you reach failure, at which point you quickly lower the weight and finish the set. This method aids in exhausting the muscles and promoting additional muscle growth.

7. **Mind-Muscle Connection:** Effective muscle growth and toning require a strong mind-muscle connection. It entails concentrating on the particular muscle being exercised and intentionally employing that muscle throughout the exercise. This method improves muscle recruitment and activation, which yields superior outcomes.

8. Recovery and correct nutrition are essential for muscle growth and toning, as is enough rest and recovery time. Ensure that your diet is well-balanced and contains adequate amounts of protein, carbs, and healthy fats to assist muscle growth and repair. The healing and growth of muscles depend on getting enough rest and sleep

CHAPTER 4

FLEXIBILITY AND BALANCE: UNLOCKING YOUR BODY'S POTENTIAL

Although they are sometimes neglected components of fitness, flexibility, and balance are crucial for general health and well-being. Increased mobility is made possible by increased flexibility, while the risk of falls and accidents is decreased by improved balance. You can gain a variety of advantages and enhance your physical performance by utilizing the flexibility and balance of your body. Let's examine the significance of balance and flexibility and learn practical methods to maximize your body's potential:

The Benefits of Flexibility

- **Increased Range of Motion:** Flexibility exercises help your joints move more freely, which makes it easier for you to move around and carry out tasks.
- **Injury Prevention:** Joints and muscles that are flexible are less likely to sustain injuries. Increased flexibility reduces the risk of injuries like joint sprains, muscle strains, and other common ailments.
- **Improvements in Posture and Alignment:** Flexibility exercises help to maintain good posture and alignment,

which lowers the risk of muscular imbalances and postural problems.

- Stretching activities improve blood flow to the muscles, assisting in their recovery after strenuous exercise and encouraging relaxation.

Strategies for Increasing Flexibility:

- **Static stretching:** Focus on feeling a gentle stretch without pain while holding a stretch for 15 to 30 seconds for a particular muscle or muscle group. Does each stretch two or three times?
- Dynamic stretching entails making slow, repeated motions that progressively widen the range of motion. Leg swings, arm circles, and walking lunges are a few examples.
- Stretching, balance, and strength exercises are used in yoga and pilates to enhance flexibility, posture, and all-around body awareness.
- **Foam rolling:** Apply pressure on tight muscles using a foam roller to relieve tension and increase flexibility.

The Benefits of Balance:

- **Fall Prevention:** Having a good balance helps us avoid falling, especially as we get older. It supports stability during regular activities and athletic endeavors.

- **Functional Movement:** Activities like walking on uneven surfaces or ascending stairs call for stability and coordination, both of which are aided by balance.
- Balance exercises work the core muscles, enhancing stability and total core strength.

Methods for Increasing Balance

- **Exercises on One Leg:** Try exercises that require you to balance on just one leg, such as single-leg squats, single-leg deadlifts, or standing with your eyes closed.
- Yoga and Tai Chi both involve flowing motions and balance poses that enhance coordination, body control, and balance.
- **Balance boards and equipment for stability training**: To test your balance and increase stability, use balance boards, stability balls, or wobble cushions.
- Exercises for proprioception Your body's capacity to perceive its location and motion in space is known as proprioception. Proprioception can be improved by exercises like standing on foam pads or doing exercises while closing your eyes.

You may maximize the potential of your body and gain a variety of advantages by including flexibility and balance exercises in your workout regimen. To prevent damage, always warm up before stretching, and begin with slow, moderate movements. Over time, gradually increase the difficulty and length of your workouts. Keep in mind to pay attention to your body and to stop if you feel pain or discomfort. Exercises for flexibility and balance should be incorporated into your routine at least two to three times a week because consistency is important. Enjoy the process of discovering new levels of flexibility and stability as you unlock your body's potential.

Embracing the significance of flexibility and balance exercises

Understanding the value of flexibility and balance training is a life-changing journey that can improve your physical performance, lower your risk of injury, and improve your general well-being. You can gain several advantages and realize the full potential of your body by including these exercises in your fitness regimen. Let's explore why doing balance and flexibility exercises is so important:

1. **Improvement of Physical Performance**
- **Greater Range of Motion:** Flexibility workouts make your muscles and joints more flexible, enhancing your range of motion. This can improve how well you perform in a variety of physical activities, including sports, dance, and even daily jobs.

- **Smooth and Efficient Movement:** Greater flexibility and balance result in movement patterns that are more fluid and effective. This will enable you to work more precisely and gracefully while also enhancing your athletic performance.

2. **Cut Back on Injury Risk:**
- Strengthening the muscles around your joints through balance exercises increases joint stability and lowers the chance of sprains and strains.
- **Improved Body Control:** Through targeted workouts, you can improve your balance and coordination and keep control over your movements, which lowers your risk of falls and other accidents.

3. **Encourage general well-being:**
- **tension Reduction:** Balance and flexibility activities, like yoga or tai chi, involve breathing exercises and mindful movements that can reduce tension, encourage relaxation, and enhance mental health.
- Better posture and alignment are made possible by these exercises, which also help to lessen muscular imbalances and the stress placed on your body's structures.
- Exercises for flexibility and balance help to improve the mind-body connection, which fosters a better understanding of your body's potential and raises your level of general body awareness.

4. **Keep your joints healthy:**

- **Joint Lubrication:** By encouraging the production of synovial fluid, which lubricates the joints and lessens friction, flexibility exercises assist preserve joint health.
- **Delayed Age-Related Decline:** Regular flexibility and balancing exercises can help avoid stiffness and improve mobility as you age by delaying age-related losses in joint flexibility.

5. **A holistic strategy for fitness**

- Strength training, aerobic workouts, and other forms of exercise should all be combined with flexibility and balance exercises to create a well-rounded fitness regimen that addresses all facets of physical fitness.
- **Exercises for Flexibility and Balance Promote Mindful Movement:** Mindful movement encourages a closer connection between your body, mind, and breath.

You may unleash your body's potential and go on a revolutionary journey toward better physical performance, fewer injuries, and greater general well-being by realizing the importance of flexibility and balancing exercises. Stretching, yoga, tai chi, or particular balance-focused activities are just a few examples of the flexibility and balancing exercises you can incorporate into your regimen. Start carefully, pay attention to your body, and add more difficult moves with time. The substantial advantages that flexibility and balance offer to your life can be experienced by embracing the process.

Enhancing mobility, preventing injuries, and improving posture

Maintaining a healthy and active lifestyle requires achieving important goals like increasing mobility, preventing injuries, and improving posture. You can go a lot closer to reaching these goals by adding particular workouts and developing mindful practices. Let's look at how increasing mobility, avoiding accidents, and correcting your posture can all contribute to your well-being:

1. **Increasing Mobility**
- A greater range of motion can be achieved with regular mobility exercises like stretching and joint mobilization. You can move more easily and carry out tasks with more ease because of this.
- Maintaining and enhancing mobility helps to maintain and improve the health and function of your joints. This can lessen joint discomfort, stiffness, and the chance of developing illnesses like arthritis.
- **Functional Movement:** Greater mobility enables you to carry out daily activities more quickly and with less effort. It assists motions like bending, reaching, and twisting, which enhances your quality of life overall.
2. **Avoiding Accidents:**
- **Flexibility and elasticity of the muscles:** Having flexible muscles lowers the risk of muscle tears and

strains during physical activity. It enables your muscles to adjust and react to rapid movements or changes in direction in an efficient manner.

- **Joint Stability:** By performing specific workouts, you can strengthen the muscles around your joints and improve stability. Through greater support and control, this helps avoid common injuries including sprains and dislocations.

- **Technique and body alignment:** Using the right form and technique when engaging in different activities, such as lifting weights or playing sports, lowers the chance of injuries brought on by poor movement patterns.

3. **Optimising Posture**

- **Spinal Alignment:** Maintaining good posture helps your spine stay in its proper position, relieving stress on your neck, shoulders, and back. It can assist in reducing discomfort and avoiding long-term posture problems.

- **Muscle Symmetry and Alignment:** Correcting muscular imbalances with activities that enhance posture can enhance muscle symmetry and alignment. This encourages improved postural support and lowers the possibility of musculoskeletal problems.

- **Positivity and Presence:** Good posture improves your appearance as a whole and exudes confidence. It may have a good effect on both how you see yourself and how others see you.

Consider adding the following exercises to your program to increase mobility, reduce injuries, and improve posture:

- Regular flexibility and stretching exercises help increase muscle suppleness and joint mobility.
- Exercises that improve general stability through strength training concentrate on the muscles supporting your joints.
- Yoga, Pilates, and tai chi are examples of mindful movement exercises that emphasize optimal alignment, body awareness, and posture.
- Make ergonomic changes to your workspace and daily routine to support good posture.
- pursuing a healthy, active lifestyle that incorporates a range of exercises that use various muscle regions and gait patterns.

You may increase your mobility, prevent injuries, and improve your posture with constant effort and a thoughtful approach, improving your overall well-being and allowing you to live a more active and pain-free life.

CHAPTER 5

THE MIND-BODY CONNECTION: EXERCISE AS A CATALYST FOR MENTAL WELL-BEING

Exploring the profound impact of exercise on mental health

Exercise acts as a catalyst for boosting mental health because of the strong mind-body link. Regular physical activity has a significant positive impact on your mental and emotional health in addition to your physical health. Let's look at some of the astonishing ways that exercise improves mental health:

1. **Mood Elevation**
- **Endorphin Release:** Endorphins, or "feel-good" hormones, are released as a result of exercise. These brain chemicals contribute to mood elevation, pain reduction, and stress reduction.
- **Reduced Stress and Anxiety:** Exercise reduces the release of stress hormones and encourages relaxation, acting as a natural stress reliever. It can ease anxiety symptoms and instill a sense of tranquility.

- **Increase in Serotonin and Dopamine:** Serotonin and dopamine are neurotransmitters linked to emotions of happiness, pleasure, and general well-being. Exercise enhances the production and availability of these neurotransmitters.

2. **Stress Reduction:**

- Exercise is an excellent way to get stress and anxiety out that has built up. It enables you to better manage stress by refocusing your attention and energy.
- **Improved Coping Mechanisms:** By boosting resilience and giving you a sense of control over difficult situations, regular exercise can help you cope with stress better.
- **Improved Memory and Mental Clarity:** Exercise encourages increased blood flow to the brain, which can improve memory and mental clarity as well as cognitive performance. Better stress management is supported as a result of this.

3. **Mental Health Issues:**

- Exercise has been demonstrated to be useful in lowering the signs and symptoms of depression and anxiety. It can improve your mood, increase your self-confidence, and give you a sense of accomplishment.
- Exercise can be used as a supplemental therapy for problems like sadness, anxiety, and even attention-deficit hyperactivity disorder (ADHD), and it has been linked to a lower risk of mental health disorders.

4. **Body image and self-esteem:**
- **Body Confidence:** Exercising regularly and reaching your fitness objectives can improve your body image and boost your self-confidence. Exercise fosters self-confidence, self-acceptance, and enjoyment of one's body.
- Participating in team sports or group exercises can offer chances for social connection, support, and a sense of belonging, all of which can have a good effect on one's self-esteem.

5. **Cognitive advantages:**
- **Increased Mental Acuity and Focus:** Regular exercise has been associated with increased cognitive function, which includes better focus, attention, and problem-solving skills.
- **Memory Improvement:** Exercise encourages the development of new brain cells, which enhances memory and learning.

To maximize exercise's positive effects on mental health:

- **Find exercises you enjoy doing:** You'll be more likely to persist with a fitness program if you find it to be fun and interesting.
- **Set attainable targets:** To feel successful and make progress, set exercise objectives that are both attainable and realistic.

- **Put consistency first:** Even if they are shorter in length, try to engage in frequent exercise sessions. Gaining the advantages of exercise for mental health requires consistency.

- **combine strength and aerobic exercise:** For maximum mental health advantages, combine aerobic exercises like jogging or swimming with strength training activities like weightlifting or bodyweight exercises.

- **Practice mindfulness:** To strengthen the mind-body connection and advance mental wellness, partake in mindful activities like yoga or tai chi.

Always remember to pay attention to your body, move at your speed, and get medical advice if you have any underlying health issues. You can benefit from exercise's incredible advantages and foster a healthy mind-body connection for a happier and healthier existence by adopting exercise as a catalyst for mental well-being.

Managing stress, improving mood, and boosting cognitive function

Maintaining total wellbeing necessitates controlling stress, elevating mood, and enhancing cognitive ability. Finding practical methods to assist our mental health in today's hectic society is essential. Fortunately, exercise provides a potent remedy to deal with these problems. Let's examine how exercising can reduce stress, elevate mood, and enhance cognitive function:

1. **Controlling Stress:**
- **Regulation of Stress Hormones:** Exercise lowers cortisol levels in the body and encourages a more balanced stress response by regulating the synthesis of stress hormones like cortisol.
- Exercise offers a channel for physically releasing tension and bottled-up stress, producing relaxation and a sensation of serenity.
- Physical exercise can serve as a mental diversion from tensions, enabling you to change your concentration and refocus your mental energy.

2. **Increasing mood**
- Exercise causes the release of endorphins, which are the brain's natural mood-enhancing substances. This can aid in reducing anxiety, despair, and mood swings in general.
- Physical exercise boosts the availability and production of serotonin and dopamine, two neurotransmitters linked to motivation, pleasure, and happiness.
- **Self-Efficacy and Confidence:** Reaching fitness milestones or going through personal development

through exercise can boost self-worth, self-efficacy, and general disposition.

3. **Enhancing Cognitive Process:**

- **Increased Blood Flow to the Brain:** Exercise stimulates blood circulation, which increases the amount of oxygen and nutrients that reach the brain, improving cognitive function and promoting brain health.

- Exercise regularly to support neuroplasticity, the brain's capacity to rearrange and create new connections. Memory, learning, and mental flexibility all benefit from this.

- **Focus and Mental Clarity:** Physical activity can promote mental clarity, increase focus, and enhance general cognitive performance.

To include exercise in your routine for stress management, mood enhancement, and cognitive function enhancement:

- **Discover activities you like:** To enhance motivation and sustainability, pick exercises that you actually enjoy.

- **Set attainable targets:** Set attainable objectives that are in line with your level of fitness and schedule to feel growth and accomplishment.

- Regularly engage in aerobic activity Aim for at least 150 minutes per week of moderate-intensity exercise or 75 minutes per week of strenuous exercise.

- Utilize strength training To improve muscle strength and general fitness, incorporate strength training exercises at least twice per week.
- Consistency is important, so make an effort to exercise regularly throughout the week to reap the rewards over time.
- Pay heed to your body's cues and avoid overexertion by listening to it. For overall health, it is imperative to get enough sleep and recover.

You can effectively control stress, elevate mood, and enhance cognitive function by adding exercise into your routine. Accept physical activity's ability to improve your mental health and open the door to a better, happier, and more balanced existence.

CAPTER 6

CUSTOMIZING YOUR FITNESS ROUTINE: DESIGNING AN EXERCISE PLAN THAT WORKS FOR YOU

Assessing your fitness goals and creating a personalized exercise regimen

The secret to reaching your fitness objectives and keeping up a sustainable fitness regimen is creating an activity plan that works for you. Every person is different, in their tastes, needs, and degrees of fitness. You can construct a workout regimen that is specifically tailored to your needs and smoothly integrates into your lifestyle. Here's how to create an exercise schedule that suits your needs:

1. **Determine Your Objectives and Fitness Level:**
- **Set Specific Goals:** Determine the goals you have for your workout program. Clarifying your goals will help your workout strategy, whether they are for weight loss,

muscular growth, bettering cardiovascular health, or general well-being.

- Assessing your level of fitness To find out where you stand, evaluate your current level of fitness. Think about things like your strength, balance, flexibility, and cardiovascular stamina. Your exercise selection and goal-setting will be aided by this evaluation.

2. **Take Your Preferences and Interests Into Account**:

- **Find Exercise Activities You Truly Enjoy:** Choose exercises that you truly enjoy. Running, swimming, dancing, cycling, or taking part in team sports are some examples. You're more likely to remain with it and maintain your motivation if you enjoy the activity.

- **Diversity and Flexibility:** To keep your regimen fresh and avoid monotony, mix up your exercises. Consider exercises that may be done in many settings as well, such as indoor or outdoor activities, based on your tastes and the resources you have at your disposal.

3. **Set definite, realistic goals:**

- Set SMART goals, which are defined as being specific, measurable, achievable, relevant, and time-bound. Instead of setting a general goal like "get fit," for instance, try "run a 5K race within three months" or "do ten push-ups without pausing."

- **Gradual Advancement:** As your level of fitness increases, gradually up the intensity, duration, or frequency of your workouts by starting with more manageable goals. This strategy lowers the possibility of injury while allowing your body to adjust.

4. **Schedule Your Workouts:**

- **Determine Your Weekly Frequency:** Choose the number of days per week that you can dedicate to working out. To allow your body to heal, strike a balance between consistency and rest days.

- **Time management:** Think about your daily plan and choose the times that suit you the most. Pick a time that you can consistently dedicate to your workouts, whether it's in the morning, during lunch, or in the evening.

- **Adapt as Required:** Be adaptable with your strategy and make adjustments as needed. Your workout regimen may need to be changed as a result of life events, injuries, or shifting goals. Be flexible and, if necessary, seek out other exercises or hobbies.

A customized fitness program must be created for long-term success and enjoyment. Keep in mind that persistence, commitment, and a positive outlook are essential. You will embark on a fitness journey that is unique to you by tailoring your workout to coincide with your objectives, interests, and skills, providing a sustainable and rewarding experience.

Tips for staying motivated and overcoming common barriers to exercise

Maintaining your enthusiasm and getting beyond typical obstacles to exercise might be difficult, but with the appropriate techniques, you can succeed. Here are some pointers to help you maintain motivation and get beyond typical workout roadblocks:

1. **Establish reasonable objectives:** Establish SMART (specific, measurable, attainable, relevant, and time-bound) fitness objectives that are both reasonable and doable. To make your goals more manageable and measurable, divide them into smaller milestones.
2. Discover Your Why Find out why you desire to workout. Reminding yourself of your motivations will help you stay dedicated and focused, whether it's to achieve a certain fitness milestone, reduce stress, or improve your health.
3. **Make Your Environment Supportive:** Surround yourself with positive, inspiring people who share your values. Join online communities that are focused on fitness, enroll in fitness classes, or locate a workout partner.
4. **Choose Exercises and Physical Activities You Truly Enjoy:** Find enjoyable activities to engage in. You're

more likely to stay motivated and look forward to your workouts if you're having fun while working out.

5. **Change Up Your Routine:** Add diversity to your workouts to prevent boredom. To keep things fresh and avoid monotony, try a variety of workout methods, change up your schedule, or discover new outdoor activities.

6. **Schedule Your Workouts:** Schedule your workouts in your calendar like you would other important appointments. Establish a schedule and try to keep to it as much as you can since consistency is important.

7. **Set Rewards:** Give yourself a treat for achieving milestones or finishing difficult workouts. Give yourself a massage, invest in new exercise equipment, or reward yourself with a nutritious treat that supports your fitness objectives.

8. Keep a log of your workouts, measurements, and accomplishments to track your progress. It can be quite motivating to see your progress documented on paper or through fitness monitoring applications, which can serve as a constant reminder of your success.

9. **Overcome Time Restraints:** If time is an issue, divide your workouts into more manageable, shorter sessions. Include physical activity in your routine by, for example, walking during your lunch break or choosing the stairs over the elevator.

10. **Be Resilient and Adaptive:** Because life is unpredictable, there may be occasions when your scheduled workouts are interrupted. Avoid giving up by being adaptable and flexible. Find other methods to be active, such as practicing bodyweight exercises when you can't make it to the gym or watching training videos at home.

11. **Make self-care a priority:** Give rest and recuperation a priority to take care of your body and mind. To avoid burnout and injury, permit yourself to get enough rest, wholesome food, and downtime.

12. Find an accountability buddy or sign up for a fitness group that will hold you responsible for your exercise schedule. Having a partner with whom to discuss your development, difficulties, and achievements can boost your motivation and support.

Keep in mind that motivation may change over time, but by putting these ideas into practice and being dedicated to your goals, you may get beyond typical obstacles and keep up a regular exercise schedule. Celebrate your successes, embrace the journey, and keep working toward a healthier and more active way of life.

CHAPTER 7

EXERCISE FOR LIFE: INTEGRATING PHYSICAL ACTIVITY INTO YOUR DAILY ROUTINE

Incorporating movement into everyday activities for long-term health benefits

A great strategy to improve long-term health is to incorporate movement into daily tasks. You can include physical activity into your everyday routine to make it more fun and sustainable. Your general health, energy levels, and well-being can all be improved by incorporating movement into daily activities. Here are some useful pointers for including movement in daily activities:

- Consider using walking or cycling as a mode of transportation for traveling small distances rather than only using a car or the public transportation system. These environmentally friendly, cost-effective, and physically active means of transportation are a great way to get around when running errands or going to work.

- **Taking Active Breaks:** Take active breaks to break up extended periods of sitting. Every hour, set a timer to serve as a reminder to get up and move around. Stretch, perform a small workout, or go for a quick stroll around your house or workplace. These little periods of mobility can assist to increase energy, enhance circulation, and counteract the harmful consequences of extended sitting.

- **include domestic duties:** Take advantage of the chance to engage in physical activity by including domestic duties. Moving while doing chores like vacuuming, sweeping, mopping, gardening, and cleaning can help you burn calories and build muscle. Make your chores fun and engaging by turning on some music.

- **Taking Part in Active Leisure:** Investigate active alternatives to sedentary leisure activities. Hike, swim, dance, play a sport, or partake in outdoor pursuits like camping or gardening. Along with encouraging physical fitness, these hobbies also offer mental and emotional renewal.

- **Choosing the Stairs:** Whenever possible, take the stairs rather than an escalator or an elevator. A great approach to use your leg muscles, enhance cardiovascular health, and burn calories is to climb stairs. Your amount of daily exercise may change significantly with one straightforward change.

- **Including Movement When Watching TV or Using Electronics:** If you find that you spend a lot of time watching TV or using electronic devices, make it a habit to include movement when you're sedentary. Do workouts like push-ups, lunges, or squats during the ad breaks. Watch your preferred television shows or movies while using a treadmill or fitness bike. You can do this to incorporate entertainment with exercise.

- Consider integrating active socializing choices rather than just meeting friends or family for food or drinks. Arrange a friendly sporting event, go on a trek together, or go biking. You'll exercise and spend time with your loved ones in addition to enjoying quality time.

- **Making Movement a Priority:** Change your perspective to move a priority in your everyday activities. Look for opportunities to be active, such as choosing an active hobby or leisure activity, taking the long way to your destination, parking farther away from the door, etc. You'll unavoidably include more physical activity in your routine if you prioritize movement.

For long-term health advantages, it is effective to incorporate movement into daily activities. Keep in mind that even the smallest adjustments can lead to a more active and healthy lifestyle. So begin today by incorporating movement into your everyday routines and relish the benefits it has on your general well-being.

CHAPTER 8

OVERCOMING CHALLENGES: STRATEGIES FOR MAINTAINING CONSISTENCY AND OVERCOMING PLATEAUS

Overcoming obstacles and staying committed to your exercise journey

When it comes to keeping up a workout routine and enjoying the long-term advantages, consistency is essential. On the other hand, obstacles and plateaus are commonplace on the journey. The good news is that you can use tactics to get around these challenges and maintain your course. The following are some sensible methods for sustaining consistency and getting past plateaus in your fitness journey:

- **Set Achievable Goals First,** set goals that are both attainable and reasonable. You'll be more motivated and laser-focused as a result. Divide your more ambitious objectives into more manageable stages. Celebrate your accomplishments along the way to keep yourself inspired to keep going.

- **Find Your Motivation:** Decide what it is that spurs you on to work out. It can be enhancing your health, increasing your energy, lowering your stress level, or reaching a certain fitness objective. When faced with obstacles or a lack of motivation, keep reminding yourself of your motivation.
- **Make a timetable:** Make a timetable that works for you by scheduling your workouts in advance. Consider these meetings with yourself as non-negotiable appointments. Find a time of day that works with your schedule and suits your level of energy. Exercise should be a top priority in your schedule since consistency is developed via regularity.
- **Change Up Your program:** When your body gets used to an exercise program, plateaus can happen. To get over this, mix up your routines by adding new exercises, training techniques, or fitness programs. This keeps your workouts interesting and challenges your body in different ways, preventing stagnation.
- **Track Your Progress:** Keep a record of your exercises, advancements, and successes. Observing your progress and the progress you have achieved can inspire you. To keep track of your exercise levels, establish goals, and

monitor your development over time, use a fitness notebook, smartphone app, or wearable fitness tracker.

- **Find a Partner for Accountability:** Having someone to hold you accountable will improve your consistency tremendously. Find a workout partner or sign up for a class or club where you can meet others who have similar interests and aspirations. Consistency can be greatly improved by supporting and encouraging one another.

- **Be Kind to Yourself and Remain Positive:** Throughout your fitness journey, practice kindness toward yourself and remain flexible. Recognize that you can experience failures or days when you lack motivation. Accept these circumstances as chances for development and adaptability. If necessary, alter your routines or attempt a different strategy, but never forget to keep going forward.

- **Set recuperation first:** Plateaus can occasionally be an indication that your body needs enough time to relax and recover. Make sure you schedule rest days into your schedule and engage in self-care activities like foam rolling, stretching, and getting enough sleep. By taking care of your body, you may recuperate as quickly as possible and avoid burnout.

- **Celebrate Your Successes:** As You Go Along, Recognize and Celebrate Your Successes. Take some time to celebrate and treat yourself when you achieve a fitness milestone, overcome a difficult situation, or see improvements in your strength or endurance. You'll remain energized and enthusiastic about continuing your trip thanks to this encouraging feedback.

Keep in mind that sustaining consistency and getting over plateaus call for tolerance for failure, tenacity, and flexibility. You may overcome obstacles, break through plateaus, and experience ongoing progress in your quest to become a healthier, fitter version of yourself by putting these techniques into practice and remaining dedicated to your fitness goals.

CHAPTER 9

THE POWER OF COMMUNITY: FINDING SUPPORT AND ACCOUNTABILITY

The benefits of exercising with others and joining fitness communities

Starting a fitness journey can be a life-changing event, but you don't have to go it alone. In terms of health and fitness, the power of community is incomparable. Finding accountability and support from people who share your goals can greatly improve your motivation, dedication, and overall performance. Here are some reasons why embracing the power of community is essential for your fitness journey, whether it be through joining a fitness group, taking part in group courses, or looking for online communities:

- **Inspiration & Motivation:** Being a part of a community exposes you to people who have like aims and goals. Observing others work toward their fitness goals can motivate and inspire you to continue on your path. Stories of success, change, and tenacity you'll hear about will inspire you to keep moving forward.

- **Accountability and commitment:** You are more likely to have a sense of responsibility to turn up and put out your best effort when you are a member of a community. You may be more motivated to stick with and dedicate yourself to your exercise regimen if you are aware that others are depending on you and supporting you. Sharing your achievements and objectives with others also makes you more responsible for achieving your own goals.

- Together, we can overcome obstacles. Every fitness path comes with its share of obstacles and failures. When you're part of a community, you have people to turn to for support when things go tough. You can seek advice, support, and compassion from your community when facing challenges. Sharing your challenges and victories with those who have traveled the same path as you can bring comfort and aid in problem-solving.

- **Fun and camaraderie:** Working out doesn't have to be a lone activity. Being a part of a community gives your workout program a social component. You can interact with people who have hobbies, interests, and objectives. Participating in group exercises, workshops, or other activities promotes camaraderie and offers a friendly atmosphere where you may have a good time while working toward your fitness objectives.

- **New Possibilities and Adventures:** You'll probably find new fitness possibilities and adventures within a community that you might not have thought of on your lonesome. The community may introduce you to exciting activities that add diversity and excitement to your fitness journey, whether it's taking part in a charity run, trying a new sport, or signing up for a fitness challenge.

- **Celebrating Milestones and Progress:** The community serves as a venue for you to recognize your accomplishments, both significant and insignificant. It can be tremendously gratifying to share your accomplishments with people who appreciate the value of your milestones, records, or progress images. Your sense of self-worth is further strengthened by the community's support and encouragement, which inspires you to do even more.

- **Long-Lasting Friendships:** The connections made within the fitness community frequently go beyond the online community or the club. Connecting with people who share your enthusiasm for health and fitness might help you form sincere friendships. In addition to creating a network of people who can continue to assist one another's growth in all areas of life, these friendships provide people with a sense of community.

You don't have to go it alone when it comes to accomplishing your fitness objectives. Accept the power of community and surround yourself with people that inspire, challenge, and uplift you. Together, you'll pave the way to a version of yourself that is stronger, healthier, and more alive. Join a group, interact with others, and discover the transformational power of finding

Harnessing the power of social support for long-term success

Gaining long-term success on your fitness quest requires harnessing the power of social support. You build a strong foundation for ongoing development when you surround yourself with a supportive network of friends, family, or like-minded people who share your commitment to health and well-being. Here are some ways that utilizing social support might help you succeed in the long run:

- **Encouragement and Accountability:** Social support offers the motivation and responsibility necessary to maintain your fitness goals. Having someone to encourage you, recognize your successes, and reaffirm your commitment keeps you committed and responsible. If you have a workout partner, a friend who is encouraging, or an online group, their support, and encouragement will greatly improve your consistency and adherence.

- **Shared Objectives and Comparable Attitudes:** Surrounding yourself with others who have comparable objectives and attitudes foster a potent atmosphere for growth. Engaging with others who share your goals for fitness and health allows you to share ideas, develop mutually beneficial techniques, and gain insight from one another's experiences. This common goal fosters a sense of community and shared knowledge that solidifies your commitment and aids in overcoming hurdles.

- Social support networks give users access to a multitude of information and tools. People in your support network might have insightful opinions, in-depth knowledge, or helpful suggestions on exercise regimens, diet plans, or recuperation approaches. You may increase your understanding and equip yourself with tools to make the most of your fitness journey by exchanging information and learning from others' experiences.

- **Motivation and emotional support:** Starting a fitness journey can be difficult at times, so having a support network is essential. The emotional support from your network can uplift your spirits, increase your confidence, and serve as a reminder of your progress when you are faced with setbacks, plateaus, or moments of uncertainty. Their inspiration and motivation turn into a driving force that aids in your perseverance during challenging times.

- **Overcoming Obstacles and Developing Resilience:** Social support can help you get beyond obstacles that could be getting in the way of your progress. Having others who understand and empathize with your troubles can provide invaluable insights and solutions for overcoming hurdles, whether they are caused by a lack of time, self-doubt, or outside difficulties. You build resilience, acquire problem-solving techniques, and become better prepared to face obstacles in the future through shared experiences and support.

- **Healthy Competition and Inspiration:** In a group of encouraging friends, healthy competition may develop, inspiring you to exert more effort. Observing others achieve success or make advancements might energize and inspire you to improve your efforts. Friendly competition can spur growth because it motivates you to set higher expectations, push your boundaries, and constantly seek progress.

- A layer of happiness and pleasure is added to your journey when you share your accomplishments and celebrate milestones with your support network. Having others recognize and applaud your achievements strengthens your sense of accomplishment and builds your confidence, whether it's accomplishing a difficult race or learning a new athletic ability.

- Social support networks developed around physical fitness and overall well-being frequently result in lifelong ties and satisfying partnerships. People become closer because of their common interests, experiences, and aspirations. These connections go beyond fitness and can improve your life in a variety of ways by giving you a sense of community, camaraderie, and a support system of like-minded people.

A revolutionary step toward long-term success on your fitness quest is harnessing the power of social support. Your motivation, knowledge, and general enjoyment of the process can be greatly improved by surrounding yourself with a supportive network of people who encourage you, inspire you, and hold you accountable. Fostering meaningful relationships and embracing the power of social support will help you live a healthier, happier, and more fulfilling life.

CONCLUSION

Embrace the Power of Regular Exercise

Exercise regularly is a potent instrument that can significantly improve your life in a variety of ways. You can benefit in a variety of ways—physical, mental, and emotional—by embracing the power of exercise. Exercise has amazing potential for everything from increasing mood and cognitive function to building muscles and improving cardiovascular health.

We have looked at the science behind exercise, examined the many physical and emotional advantages it brings, and offered tips for incorporating it into your daily routine throughout this journey. Goal-setting, conquering challenges, and getting help along the way have all been covered.

Take action right away and start making fitness a top priority in your life. Start by evaluating your fitness objectives and creating a customized training schedule that suits your requirements and interests. Discovering activities you enjoy, making use of social support, and celebrating your accomplishments will help you stay motivated. Utilize a growth mentality and patience to get through obstacles and plateaus.

Keep in mind that regular exercise has benefits outside of scheduled workouts. Adopt an active lifestyle by including movement in your daily routine and looking for opportunities to exercise throughout the day. Be aware of your body's requirements, take care of yourself, and pay attention to any indications it provides you.

Know that you are capable of doing incredible things as you set out on your trip. You are investing in yourself with each step you take toward a fitter, healthier, and more balanced lifestyle. Accept the power of consistent exercise and allow it to bring out the best in you.

So, lace up your shoes, don your gym gear, and start your amazing journey. You can change your life. Take advantage of it, embrace it, and allow the power of consistent exercise to lead you to a healthier, happier self in the future.

Reflecting on the transformative power of exercise on overall health

Regular physical activity is not just a task to cross off a to-do list as it becomes obvious as we consider the transforming impact of exercise on overall health. It catalyzes transformation and a starting point for a life full of vigor, fortitude, and well-being.

We have investigated the science of exercise throughout our journey, learning how it improves both our physical and mental health. We have seen firsthand the amazing advantages it offers, from enhancing cardiovascular fitness and muscle definition to stress reduction and improved cognitive function. We've seen time and time again how effective exercise is in helping us live longer, healthier lives.

But exercise has more meaning than just the bodily benefits. It demonstrates the tenacity and power of the human soul. It teaches us self-control, tenacity, and the ability to push past our comfort zones. We are pushed to stretch beyond our comfort zones and unlock new levels of our potential.

Exercising has transform effects that go far beyond the running track or the gym. Every element of our life is affected by it, including our relationships, our jobs, and our general sense of self. Regular physical activity helps us develop a self-care mindset and makes our health a priority. As we exercise more, we become more in tune with our bodies, paying attention to their requirements and taking care of them.

Exercise is not a treatment that works for everyone. It is a personal journey that is particular to each person. We must identify the pursuits that make us happy, stoke our passion, and fit with our inclinations. What matters is that we move our bodies and respect their intrinsic yearning for movement, whether that be through a rigorous workout, yoga, a trip in the woods, or a dancing class.

Let's not overlook the significance of balance as we consider the transforming potential of exercise. It is not about striving for an elusive standard of perfection or pushing ourselves to the point of fatigue. Finding a healthy rhythm that nourishes our bodies and minds will enable us to flourish in all facets of life.

In light of this, keep in mind that there are more benefits to regular exercise than just the physical ones as you start your path. It is about internal change, the sense of empowerment, and the forthcoming resurgence of vigor.

Accept the positive effects of exercise. Accept the pleasure of movement. Make it a regular part of your life to see the amazing effects it has on your general health and well-being. You deserve to have a life that is full of vigor, energy, and vibrancy. Everything begins with one action, one exercise, and a dedication to oneself.

Embracing a lifelong commitment to physical activity for a healthier, happier you

Your future will be shaped by your decision to embrace a lifelong commitment to physical activity, which will help you become a healthier, happier version of yourself. It is a long-term investment in your well-being and quality of life, rather than focusing on transient trends or short-lived ambitions.

Making regular physical activity a part of your daily routine will enhance your health for the rest of your life. Regular exercise benefits your mind and spirit as much as your physical health. It becomes a pillar of your general well-being and gives you the vigor, vigor, and energy to thrive in all facets of life.

When you decide to engage in regular physical activity, you set out on a quest for personal growth. You transcend your expectations as you find your hidden qualities and abilities. You acquire self-control, tenacity, and a sense of accomplishment that transcends fitness.

A lifelong dedication to physical activity also promotes a healthy relationship with your body. You learn to pay attention to its cues, respect its boundaries, and pay attention to what it requires. This link turns into a compass, enabling you to make decisions that promote your health and well-being.

Keep in mind that no one strategy works for everyone on this trip. Find the things you enjoy doing, whether it's yoga, hiking, cycling, swimming, or any other activity. Accept variation, enabling yourself to experiment with many styles of movement to find what speaks to you. Finding activities you truly enjoy is the key to increasing your motivation and integrating exercise into your daily.

It's critical to approach your commitment to exercise with tolerance and compassion. Recognize that despite the ups and downs along the journey, every advance is a success in and of itself. No matter how little your development may be, acknowledge it and keep in mind that consistency is the key. Remind yourself of the long-term advantages and how much better you always feel after moving your body, even on days when motivation is low.

Finally, be aware of the strength of support and community. Do your best to surround yourself with people who share your commitment to health and well-being. Find a workout partner, sign up for a fitness class, or take part in group activities. You will be inspired and motivated by the support, friendship, and shared experiences, which will make the journey more satisfying and pleasurable.

Adopting a lifelong commitment to physical activity is an investment in your future self, not simply in the here and now. You are laying a strong foundation for a life full of vigor, vitality, and happiness by placing a high priority on your health. Take action now and let your dedication to exercise help you become a healthier, happier version of yourself—one who flourishes in body, mind, and spirit.

THANK YOU FOR CHOOSING US.

We Appreciate Your Kind Support And We Hope You Got Something Out Of It.

If You Enjoy This Book, It Will Be Great To <u>Leave a Review On Amazon</u>. It Means a Lot To Us.

ENJOY OUR SERVICES.